THRIVING WITH TLC

A COMPREHENSIVE GUIDE TO THE THERAPEUTIC LIFESTYLE CHANGES DIET

CYRIL LAKES

Contents

CHAPTER ONE

INTRODUCTION

The National Cholesterol Education Program (NCEP) of the National Institutes of Health created the heart-healthy Therapeutic Lifestyle Changes (TLC) diet. Its goal is to lower the risk of heart disease by emphasizing dietary and lifestyle adjustments. In order to promote heart health, the TLC diet places an emphasis on foods that are low in cholesterol, trans fat, and saturated fat while also encouraging a balanced dietary consumption.

The TLC diet aims to improve cardiovascular wellbeing in general in addition to lowering cholesterol levels. It highlights how crucial it is to keep a healthy weight, exercise frequently, and develop other heart-healthy behaviors.

People who follow the TLC diet can lower their risk of heart disease, stroke, and other cardiovascular disorders and significantly improve their cholesterol levels. The diet is sustainable and ideal for long-term adherence because it is adaptable to individual preferences and nutritional needs.

We'll go over the main ideas of the TLC diet, its advantages for health, suggested foods, methods for organizing meals, and advice on how to incorporate heart-healthy routines into everyday life in this book. The TLC diet can be a useful tool for reaching your wellness objectives, whether your aim is to lower your cholesterol or improve your general cardiovascular health.

A Summary of the TLC Diet

The National Cholesterol Education Program (NCEP) of the National Institutes of Health created the heart-healthy Therapeutic Lifestyle Changes (TLC) diet. Its purpose is to lower the risk of heart disease and lower hypercholesterolemia. The TLC diet emphasizes dietary modifications and the adoption of heart-healthy lifestyle practices.

Fundamental Ideas of the TLC Diet:

Cutting Down on Saturated Fat and Cholesterol: The TLC diet places a strong emphasis on cutting back on the consumption of foods high in cholesterol and saturated fat because these can increase levels of LDL cholesterol, the "bad" cholesterol linked to heart disease.

Increasing Fiber and Whole Grains: The diet promotes the eating of whole grains, legumes, fruits, and vegetables as well as other foods high in fiber. These meals support heart health by lowering LDL cholesterol levels.

Selecting Lean Proteins: To assist lower cholesterol and minimize intake of saturated fat, lean protein sources including fish, chicken, legumes, and tofu are favored over high-fat meats.

Restricting Trans Fats and Refined Sugars: Due to their potential to elevate low-density lipoprotein (LDL) cholesterol and increase the risk of heart disease, foods containing trans fats and refined sugars should be avoided.

Portion Size Monitoring: Restricting portion sizes helps you keep a healthy weight, which supports heart health, and manage your calorie consumption.

Including Regular Exercise: The TLC diet places a strong emphasis on the value of regular exercise for maintaining general cardiovascular health. On most days of the week, try to get in at least 30 minutes of moderate-intensity exercise.

Important Elements of the TLC Diet:

Fruits and veggies: Try to make your meals and snacks consist of a range of vibrant fruits and veggies. These are high in fiber and low in calories, plus they supply vital vitamins, minerals, and antioxidants.

Whole Grains: To enhance fiber consumption and support heart health, go for whole grain products like brown rice, quinoa, oats, whole wheat bread, and whole grain pasta.

Lean Proteins: Choose foods high in lean protein, such as fish, lentils, skinless chicken, tofu, and lean meat portions. Limit your consumption of processed and high-fat meats.

Good Fats: Incorporate moderate amounts of foods high in healthy fats, such as avocados, nuts, seeds, and olive oil. These fats can promote heart health and lower cholesterol.

Low-Fat Dairy: To cut back on your consumption of saturated fat, opt for low-fat or fat-free dairy products. These consist of cheese, yogurt, and milk.

Reduce Saturated and Trans Fats: Eat less fatty meats, full-fat dairy products, fried foods, and commercially baked items, among other foods high in saturated and trans fats.

Watch Sodium Intake: Reducing sodium intake can be achieved by avoiding highly processed foods, which are frequently rich in sodium, and by selecting low- or no-sodium options.

Moderate Alcohol Consumption: Use moderation when consuming alcohol if you decide to do so. For women, the daily limit is one drink, and for men, it is two drinks.

The TLC diet is a heart-healthy eating plan that emphasizes dietary adjustments and lifestyle alterations to lower high cholesterol and the risk of heart disease. The TLC diet can assist people in improving their general well-being and cardiovascular health by placing an emphasis on nutrient-rich foods, minimizing harmful fats and sweets, and encouraging frequent physical activity.

Recognizing the Fundamentals of the TLC Diet

It is imperative to comprehend the tenets of the TLC (Therapeutic Lifestyle Changes) diet in order to execute this heart-healthy eating regimen with efficiency. Through dietary changes and lifestyle adjustments, the TLC diet is specifically designed to lower high cholesterol levels and lower the risk of heart disease. Here's a closer look at the TLC diet's main tenets:

1. Cutting Back on Dietary Cholesterol and Saturated Fat:

Diminish Saturated Fat: Saturated fats can elevate LDL cholesterol levels, which increases the risk of heart disease. They are mostly present in animal products like meat and dairy as well as in some plant-based oils like coconut oil. Less than 7% of daily calories should come from saturated fat, according to the TLC diet.

Handling Dietary Cholesterol: Animal-based foods like dairy, meat, and eggs contain cholesterol. The TLC diet suggests consuming no more than 200 milligrams of cholesterol per day, even though cholesterol in food has less of an effect on blood cholesterol levels than saturated fat.

2. Boosting Insoluble Fiber:

Stress Soluble Fiber: Soluble fiber, which may be found in foods such as fruits, vegetables, grains, barley, and oats, helps decrease LDL cholesterol levels by binding to and eliminating cholesterol from the body through the digestive tract. Consuming foods high in soluble fiber is encouraged by the TLC diet in order to enhance heart health.

3. Including Stanols and Plant Sterols:

Add Plant Sterols and Stanols: These naturally occurring plant-based substances have the ability to reduce LDL cholesterol levels. They function by preventing the intestines from absorbing cholesterol. The TLC diet suggests including items fortified with plant sterol and stanol, such orange juice and some margarines, in the diet.

4. Developing a Heart-Healthy Dietary Routine:

Emphasis on Whole Foods: The TLC diet advocates consuming a diet high in fruits, vegetables, whole grains, lean meats, healthy fats, and minimally processed whole foods. Essential nutrients and phytonutrients that promote heart health are found in these foods.

Moderate Portion proportions: Keeping a healthy weight and regulating calorie intake need careful attention to portion proportions. To promote general health and wellbeing, the TLC diet promotes portion control and mindful eating.

5. Encouragement of Lifestyle Adjustments:

Frequent Physical Activity: The TLC diet highlights the value of regular physical activity for heart health in addition to food modifications. Most days of the week, try to get in at least 30 minutes of moderate-intensity exercise to assist improve cardiovascular fitness and lower LDL cholesterol levels.

Sustaining a Healthy Weight: Heart health depends on achieving and sustaining a healthy weight. The TLC diet encourages people to take up lifestyle practices like consistent exercise and a well-balanced food that help them maintain their weight.

Through dietary changes, lifestyle adjustments, and heart-healthy practices, the TLC diet aims to lower high cholesterol levels and the risk of heart disease. The TLC diet offers a holistic approach to supporting cardiovascular health by lowering dietary cholesterol and saturated fat, increasing soluble fiber consumption, integrating plant sterols and stanols, adopting a heart-healthy eating pattern, and encouraging lifestyle adjustments.

The TLC (Therapeutic Lifestyle Changes) diet's dietary guidelines are intended to assist people in lowering high cholesterol and lowering their risk of heart disease. Following these recommendations entails altering your diet in ways that will strengthen your heart. The TLC diet's main dietary recommendations are as follows:

1. Don't Eat Too Much Saturated Fat:

Reduce Consumption: Cut back on foods high in saturated fats, such as palm and coconut oils, full-fat dairy products, butter, lard, and fatty meat cuts.

Select Leaner Options: Go for lean protein sources such as fish, tofu, skinless chicken, lentils, and lean meat cuts. To cut down on saturated fat intake, trim visible fat from meat and remove the skin from poultry.

2. Lower Cholesterol in Diet:

Limit Intake: Restrict your intake of items high in cholesterol from the diet, like organ meats, egg yolks, and high-fat dairy products.

Watch Portion Sizes: If you're eating items high in cholesterol, like eggs, try to limit your portion sizes and be aware of how much cholesterol you're getting overall during the day.

3. Boost the Soluble Fiber:

Eat Soluble Fiber-Rich Foods: Include foods high in soluble fiber in your diet, such as fruits, vegetables, grains, beans, lentils, and oats.

Eat Whole Grains: To increase fiber consumption and promote heart health, choose whole grain products such whole wheat bread, brown rice, quinoa, and whole grain pasta.

4. Eat Stanols and Plant Sterols:

Add Fortified Foods: Include foods like yogurt drinks, orange juice, and some margarines that have been fortified with plant sterols and stanols in your diet.

CHAPTER TWO

Consume the appropriate servings of foods fortified with plant sterols or stanols as part of your daily diet to help lower your LDL cholesterol levels.

5. Refined carbs and added sugars should be avoided.

Minimize Intake: Restrict your intake of sugary drinks, candies, pastries, and white bread, as well as other meals and beverages that are high in refined carbs and added sugars.

Select Whole Food Sources: To get your carbs, choose whole foods like fruits, vegetables, whole grains, and legumes. These foods also include fiber and other important nutrients.

6. Regulate the Size of the Portion:

Be Aware of Portions: To prevent overindulging and control calorie intake, be mindful of portion sizes.

Use Smaller dishes: You may manage portion sizes and avoid overindulging by using smaller dishes and bowls.

7. Keep an eye on your sodium intake:

Limit Sodium: Cut back on your consumption of sodium by making low- or no-sodium food choices and using less salt in the kitchen and at the table.

Read Labels: Look up the sodium level of foods on labels and, if you can, select ones with less salt.

Individuals can lower their cholesterol, lessen their risk of heart disease, and enhance their overall cardiovascular health by adhering to the TLC diet's nutritional recommendations. People can develop a heart-healthy eating pattern that promotes long-term wellness by concentrating on reducing their intake of saturated fat and dietary cholesterol, increasing their intake of soluble fiber, consuming plant sterols and stanols, selecting nutrient-dense foods, managing portion sizes, and keeping an eye on their sodium intake.

Although the TLC (Therapeutic Lifestyle Changes) diet has several health advantages, its main goals are to reduce the risk of heart disease and improve cardiovascular health. The TLC diet can significantly improve general health by focusing on heart-healthy food choices and lifestyle adjustments. The TLC diet offers the following main health benefits:

1. Reduced Levels of Cholesterol:

Decrease in LDL Cholesterol: Often known as "bad" cholesterol, low-density lipoprotein (LDL) cholesterol is the target of the TLC diet. The TLC diet lowers LDL cholesterol levels, which is important for heart health, by consuming more soluble fiber and plant sterols/stanols and consuming less saturated fats and dietary cholesterol.

2. Reduced Heart Disease Risk:

Cardiovascular Protection: The risk of heart disease, including coronary artery disease, heart attack, and stroke, can be considerably decreased by lowering LDL cholesterol levels and implementing heart-healthy dietary and lifestyle choices. The TLC diet can help protect the heart generally since it emphasizes heart-healthy eating habits and lifestyle changes.

3. Enhanced Regulation of Blood Pressure:

Reduced Blood Pressure: Adhering to the TLC diet may result in better management of blood pressure. People may see drops in blood pressure by focusing on whole meals high in minerals like potassium, magnesium, and fiber and consuming less salt. This lowers the risk of heart disease and stroke.

4. Controlling Weight:

Support for Weight Loss and Maintenance: The TLC diet restricts high-calorie, processed foods and promotes the use of nutrient-dense, low-calorie foods including fruits, vegetables, whole grains, and lean proteins. This method can assist people in reaching and maintaining a healthy weight, which is crucial for maintaining general health and preventing heart disease.

5. Enhanced Regulation of Blood Sugar:

Stabilized Blood Sugar Levels: The TLC diet's focus on whole, minimally processed foods can assist to enhance insulin sensitivity and stabilize blood sugar levels. Those who have type 2 diabetes or are at risk for the disease will benefit most from this since it can help control blood sugar levels and lower the risk of complications from the disease.

6. General Wellness and Health:

Promotion of General Wellness: The TLC diet encourages the consumption of a nutrient-dense, well-balanced diet that includes important vitamins, minerals, antioxidants, and other health-promoting substances. The TLC diet improves mood, energy, and quality of life by promoting general health and wellbeing.

Numerous health advantages of the TLC diet include reduced blood pressure, heart disease risk, cholesterol, assistance for weight management, stable blood sugar, and enhancement of general health and wellbeing. The TLC diet can help people dramatically improve their cardiovascular health and general quality of life by encouraging them to make heart-healthy food choices and lifestyle changes.

Getting the TLC Diet Started

Beginning the TLC (Therapeutic Lifestyle Changes) diet entails gradually changing one's food and way of living in order to lower cholesterol and promote heart health. The following steps will assist you in beginning the TLC diet:

1. Evaluate Your Diet Right Now:

Take Stock: Assess your present eating patterns and pinpoint areas in need of development. Make a list of all the things you frequently eat that are rich in cholesterol, saturated fat, and refined carbohydrates.

2. Establish sensible objectives:

Set Goals: Decide what your health objectives are, such as reducing cholesterol, strengthening your heart, or reaching a healthier weight. Establish measurable objectives that are in line with the TLC diet's tenets.

3. Recognize the TLC Dietary Principles:

Learn about the main tenets of the TLC diet, such as consuming soluble fiber, consuming plant sterols and stanols, minimizing saturated fat and dietary cholesterol, managing portion sizes, and keeping an eye on sodium intake.

4. Modify Your Diet:

Emphasize entire Foods: Include entire, minimally processed foods such as fruits, vegetables, whole grains, lean meats, and healthy fats in your diet. These foods promote heart health and offer vital nutrients.

Minimize Saturated Fat: Restrict the amount of foods high in saturated fats that you eat, such as butter, tropical oils, full-fat dairy products, and fatty meats. Select low-fat dairy products and lean protein sources in its place.

Reducing your intake of foods high in dietary cholesterol, such as organ meats, egg yolks, and high-fat dairy products, is one way to lower your cholesterol levels. Lean beef and poultry cuts should be used, as should egg whites or egg replacements.

Boost Soluble Fiber: Include foods high in soluble fiber in your diet, like fruits, vegetables, grains, beans, lentils, and oats. These meals promote heart health by lowering LDL cholesterol levels.

Include Plant Sterols and Stanols: To help reduce LDL cholesterol levels, include foods fortified with plant sterols and stanols, such as some margarines, orange juice, and yogurt drinks.

5. Use Portion Control Techniques:

Be Aware of Portions: To prevent overindulging and control calorie intake, be mindful of portion sizes. Employ smaller bowls and plates to help manage portion sizes and avoid overindulging.

6. Keep an eye on your sodium intake:

Limit Sodium: Cut back on your consumption of sodium by making low- or no-sodium food choices and using less salt in the kitchen and at the table. To detect high-sodium foods and select lower-sodium substitutes, read food labels.

7. Include Exercise:

Keep Moving: Try to get in at least 30 minutes a day, most days of the week, of moderate-intense physical activity. Take part in your favorite hobbies, like dancing, walking, cycling, swimming, or swimming, to promote heart health and general wellbeing.

8. Seek Assistance:

Recruit Support: To get more help and accountability, discuss your goals with friends, family, or a healthcare provider. Think about getting advice from a nutritionist or qualified dietitian, or consider joining a support group.

9. Track Development:

Track Your Progress: To keep an eye on your development throughout time, keep a record of your dietary decisions, degree of physical activity, and cholesterol readings. Celebrate your successes and adapt as necessary to keep moving toward your objectives.

Beginning the TLC diet entails introducing exercise, controlling portion sizes, seeking out support from others, and gradually altering one's diet. You may lower your cholesterol, boost heart health, and improve your general well-being by adhering to the TLC diet's tenets and forming heart-healthy habits.

Easy-to-follow Recipes & Dinner Ideas

It might be more fun and sustainable to follow the Therapeutic Lifestyle Changes (TLC) diet if you include TLC-friendly dishes and meal ideas in your diet. To get you started, consider these delectable and heart-healthy meal ideas and recipes:

For breakfast:

To make oatmeal with fresh berries, cook rolled oats in water or skim milk, then top with ground flaxseeds, honey, or maple syrup, and fresh berries (strawberries, blueberries, or raspberries).

Vegetable Omelet: Beat eggs and egg whites together, then cook with diced tomatoes, onions, bell peppers, and spinach in a nonstick skillet. Accompany with whole grain bread.

Greek Yogurt Parfait: To add crunch, layer sliced bananas, mixed berries, and low-fat Greek yogurt with chopped almonds or granola.

Lunch:

Quinoa salad with veggies and chickpeas: Mix cooked quinoa with diced cucumbers, cherry tomatoes, canned chickpeas, chopped parsley, and olive oil, lemon juice, tahini, and garlic.

Grilled Chicken Salad: Slice thinly a lean chicken breast that has been baked or grilled. Combine with cucumber, cherry tomatoes, sliced avocado, mixed greens, and a balsamic vinaigrette dressing.

Lentils, chopped tomatoes, carrots, celery, onions, and garlic can all be combined to make a filling soup. For taste, add herbs like bay leaves and thyme.

Dinner is

Roasted Vegetables with Baked fish: Drizzle fish fillets with olive oil, garlic, and herbs, and bake until flaky. Accompany with roasted veggies like cauliflower, broccoli, and carrots.

Turkey Chili: Diced tomatoes, kidney beans, onions, bell peppers, and chili spices can all be used to make a lean version of turkey chili. Garnish with chopped green onions and a dollop of low-fat Greek yogurt.

Stir-fry a mixture of vibrant veggies, such as carrots, bell peppers, broccoli, snap peas, and mushrooms, with a tiny bit of olive oil and low-sodium soy sauce. Serve with quinoa or brown rice.

Munchies:

Mixed Nuts: For a heart-healthy snack, eat a tiny handful of unsalted mixed nuts, such as cashews, walnuts, and almonds.

Hummus-Dipped Vegetable Sticks: For a wholesome and filling snack, dunk sliced bell peppers, cucumber, carrot, and cherry tomatoes in hummus.

Almond butter on Apple Slices: Almond butter provides a delightful blend of natural sweetness, fiber, and healthy fats on apple slices.

Sweets:

Fruit salad is a cool and naturally sweet dessert choice. Combine a variety of fresh fruits, such as strawberries, pineapple, grapes, and kiwi.

Baked Apples: Hollow out the cores of the apples and stuff them with oats, cinnamon, and a little honey or maple syrup. Bake till soft, then serve hot.

Dark Chocolate-Covered Strawberries: For a rich but heart-healthy treat, dunk fresh strawberries into melted dark chocolate and refrigerate.

These nutrient-dense and heart-healthy dishes and meal ideas are perfect for anyone on a TLC-friendly journey to improved cardiovascular health. Try varying the flavors and ingredients in your meals to keep them interesting and fulfilling while adhering to the TLC diet guidelines.

Advice for Meal Planning and Grocery Shopping

Meal planning and grocery buying are essential to adhering to the TLC (Therapeutic Lifestyle Changes) diet. Here are some pointers to make meal prep easier and help you shop at the grocery store:

Tips for Grocery Shopping:

Plan Ahead: Before you go to the grocery shop, make a weekly meal plan. You may stay organized and refrain from impulsive purchases by doing this.

Make a list of the things you'll need for the meals you have planned and follow it to prevent buying extraneous stuff.

Shop the Periphery: Concentrate on your grocery shopping near the store's periphery, where you can discover whole grains, dairy products, fresh produce, and lean proteins. Spend as little time as possible on the aisles, which are filled with processed and unhealthy items.

Select entire Foods: Whenever feasible, choose entire, minimally processed foods. Make sure to choose lean meat, chicken, fish, whole grains, low-fat dairy products, and fresh produce.

Read Labels: Go through food labels carefully and select items that are low in sodium, cholesterol, trans fat, and saturated fat. Seek products with few ingredients and steer clear of those with unhealthy additives and extra sugar.

Stock Up on basics: Make sure your cupboard is full of TLC-friendly basics like olive oil, nuts, seeds, canned beans, canned tomatoes, whole grains (brown rice, quinoa, and oats), and herbs and spices.

Include Plant Sterols: To help reduce LDL cholesterol, look for foods like some margarines, orange juice, and yogurt drinks that have been fortified with plant sterols and stanols.

Tips for Preparing Meals:

Prepare Ingredients Ahead of Time: Take some time to prepare ingredients in advance, including cleaning and cutting veggies, cooking grains, and marinating meats. Throughout the week, food preparation will be quicker and simpler as a result.

Cook in Bulk: Make bigger batches of food and freeze it for later use. By doing this, you can ensure that you have wholesome options available even on busy days.

Use Heart-Healthy Cooking Techniques: Opt for low-fat sautéing, baking, steaming, and grilling as heart-healthy cooking techniques. Steer clear of frying and using a lot of butter or oil.

Try Adding Flavor to Your Foods Without Relying on Too Much Salt, Sugar, or Bad Fats: Try adding flavor to your food with herbs, spices, citrus juices, and vinegar.

CHAPTER THREE

Meal and snack prep: Make ahead and package meals and snacks to bring to work, school, or other events. Having wholesome options close at hand can aid in reducing impulsive eating.

How to Store Leftovers: To preserve freshness and reduce food waste, store leftovers in the freezer or refrigerator in airtight containers. Put a date on containers so you can monitor their freshness.

Remain Organized: To expedite meal preparation, keep your kitchen tidy and orderly. Make sure you have all the pots and pans, cooking tools, and supplies on hand.

These meal planning and grocery shopping suggestions will help you make the TLC diet more sustainable and manageable. Making a plan, selecting nutrient-dense foods, and cooking in preparation will help you in your endeavors to reduce cholesterol and enhance cardiovascular health.

Eating Out and Social Events

Following the TLC (Therapeutic Lifestyle Changes) diet might make dining out and social gatherings difficult, but with a little preparation and awareness, you can handle these circumstances and still abide by heart-healthy guidelines. The following advice can help you manage social events and eating out while following the TLC diet:

Eating Outside:

Investigate Restaurants: Look up menu items that fit the TLC diet online before to going out to eat. Seek out restaurants that have a selection of fully prepared, fresh foods and dishes that may be customized.

Request Modifications: Do not be afraid to request menu item changes to make them more TLC-friendly from your waitress. Ask for steamed or roasted veggies as a side dish, grilled or baked alternatives instead of fried ones, and ask for dressings and sauces on the side.

Make A Wise Choice: When placing your order, give priority to dishes with lots of vegetables and whole grains, as well as lean protein options like grilled chicken, turkey, or fish. Steer clear of fried or highly processed foods, creamy sauces, and meats with a high fat content.

Regulate Portion Sizes: The serving sizes at restaurants are frequently greater than what you would serve yourself at home. If you are dining with someone, think about splitting an entree or ordering a to-go box so you can divide out half of your meal before you even start eating.

Be Aware of Extras: Extras like bread baskets, appetizers, and alcoholic drinks can increase the amount of calories, sodium, and saturated fat in your dinner. Therefore, be aware of these additions. Limit these extras or go for a healthy option, such as an appetizer consisting of vegetables or a side salad.

Social Events:

Plan Ahead: Have a balanced, TLC-friendly dinner in advance if you know you'll be attending a social gathering where food will be provided. This can lessen appetite and stop overindulging in unhealthy foods.

Bring a Dish: At social events, volunteer to bring a dish that is suitable for TLC to share. This guarantees that you'll always have at least one heart-healthy alternative on hand and introduces others to delectable foods that promote heart health.

When seated at a buffet or potluck-style dinner, try to eat in moderation by starting with a plate full of fruits, vegetables, and lean proteins. Treat yourself to small servings of less nutritious or higher-calorie foods.

Prioritize Socializing: Make time with friends and family a priority during social gatherings rather than letting food take center stage. Take part in non-food-related activities together, including taking a stroll, playing games, or taking up a hobby.

Be Adaptable: Although it's crucial to follow heart-healthy guidelines as closely as possible, it's acceptable to periodically reward yourself and enjoy exceptional foods in moderation. Maintain equilibrium and adaptability in your social dining strategy.

Social gatherings and eating out can be pleasurable even when adhering to the TLC diet. Planning ahead, making informed decisions, and exercising moderation will help you deal with these circumstances with assurance and maintain your focus on heart-healthy eating practices. It all comes down to finding a balance and ways to enjoy food without compromising your general health and wellbeing.

Including Exercise and Physical Activity

Including exercise and physical activity in your routine is crucial to the TLC (Therapeutic Lifestyle Changes) diet and can help decrease cholesterol and improve cardiovascular health. The following advice can help you make exercise and physical activity a part of your daily routine:

1. Establish sensible objectives:

Start Small: Set small, manageable objectives for yourself, such exercising for 30 minutes a day, most days of the week, at a moderate level. As you grow more accustomed to working out, you lengthen and intensify your sessions.

2. Select Pleasure-Seeking Activities:

Discover Your Passion: Opt for physical pursuits and workouts that you find enjoyable and eager to engage in. Exercise routines that include things you enjoy can be more fun and long-lasting, whether the activities include sports, walking, cycling, swimming, dancing, or any combination of these.

3. Keep Moving During the Day:

Move More: Seek ways to add extra movement to your daily schedule in order to raise your level of daily exercise. Choose the stairs over the elevator, park further away from your destination, and go for quick walks while you're on the job.

4. Plan Frequent Exercise Times:

Make Exercise a Priority: Set aside time each day or week for exercise, and regard this as a non-negotiable appointment. To maintain a healthy lifestyle and profit from physical activity, consistency is essential.

5. Adapt Your Exercises:

Variety is Key: To keep things fresh and avoid monotony, mix up your routine with a range of physical activities and exercises. Experiment with various regimens, including group fitness courses, strength training, cardio, and flexibility exercises.

6. Establish Clear Objectives:

Monitor Your Progress: As you work out and increase your step count, run a given distance, or lift larger weights, set clear, quantifiable objectives for yourself. Monitor your development over time and acknowledge your successes.

7. Warm Up and Dissipate:

Put Safety First: To prepare your body for exercise and lower the chance of damage, warm up before every session. Stretch afterward to increase range of motion and aid in muscle repair.

8. Pay Attention to Your Body:

Be Aware: Observe your body's sensations both during and after physical activity. Reduce the volume or intensity of your exercises if you feel pain or discomfort, and seek medical advice if necessary.

9. Drink plenty of water and feed your body:

Nutrition and Hydration: To stay hydrated, drink a lot of water prior to, during, and after exercise. To promote energy levels and muscle recovery, feed your body a diet rich in a balance of carbohydrates, protein, and healthy fats.

10. Obtain Assistance:

Accountability and Motivation: To offer accountability and motivation, look for a workout partner, enroll in a fitness program, or engage with a personal trainer. Having encouragement and support can help you stick to your fitness regimen.

Including exercise and physical activity in your routine is a crucial component of the TLC diet and will help decrease cholesterol and improve cardiovascular health. You may create a long-lasting fitness regimen that benefits your general wellbeing by prioritizing safety, choosing enjoyable activities, setting reasonable goals, and remaining consistent. Always pay attention to your body, acknowledge your accomplishments, and relish the numerous advantages of leading an active lifestyle.

Tracking Development and Making Modifications

Achieving your health objectives and successfully implementing the TLC (Therapeutic Lifestyle Changes) diet require tracking your progress and making necessary adjustments along the way. The following advice will help you keep a close eye on your development and make the required corrections:

1. Track Your Cholesterol Levels Frequently:

Arrange Follow-Up Tests: To track your development over time, work with your healthcare practitioner to arrange routine cholesterol tests. Your total cardiovascular health as well as variations in your LDL (low-density lipoprotein) cholesterol levels will be evaluated by these tests.

Monitor Changes: To monitor changes and spot trends over time, keep track of your weight, blood pressure, cholesterol levels, and other pertinent health indicators.

2. Evaluate Eating Behaviors:

Keep a Food Journal: To monitor your eating patterns, including what you eat, how much you consume, and when you eat, keep a thorough food journal. This can assist you in seeing trends, identifying problem areas, and maintaining accountability for your dietary objectives.

Examine Nutrient Intake: Make sure you're getting enough nutrients while adhering to the TLC diet by evaluating your nutrient intake. In order to receive individualized advice and recommendations, think about speaking with a licensed dietitian or nutritionist.

3. Track Your Exercise:

Track Your Exercise Sessions: Maintain a record of your workouts, including the kind, length, and intensity of each. This will enable you to track your development over time and maintain accountability for your fitness objectives.

Evaluate Your Fitness Levels: As you advance, make sure to periodically evaluate your level of fitness and establish new objectives. To monitor your progress, think about include fitness evaluations like strength, flexibility, and cardiovascular endurance testing.

4. Pay Attention to Your Body:

Pay Attention to How You Feel: Become aware of your physical, mental, and emotional well-being by tuning in to your body. Take note of any shifts in your mood, energy level, quality of sleep, and general well-being as these might offer important clues about your progress.

Handle Difficulties: Take the initiative to deal with any difficulties or roadblocks you come across. If you have trouble keeping up your workout regimen or adhering to the TLC diet, recognize possible roadblocks and devise solutions.

5. Make the Required Changes:

Review and Modify Your Objectives: Evaluate your progress and goals on a regular basis to see if any modifications are required. If you're not getting the results you want or you feel like you're plateauing, think about changing your strategy, reevaluating your objectives, or getting more help.

Try Different Things: Try making little adjustments to your food, workout regimen, or way of life to see how they affect your development. This may be experimenting with different dishes, changing up your exercise routine, or learning stress-reduction strategies.

6. Seek Advice and Assistance:

Seek Advice from competent specialists: For individualized information and recommendations, consult a registered dietitian, your healthcare practitioner, or other competent specialists. When necessary, they can provide support, keep an eye on your development, and modify your plan accordingly.

Participate in Supportive Communities: Make connections with people who are pursuing comparable health objectives or the TLC diet to get accountability, support, and encouragement.

Participate in online networks for wellbeing, support groups, or to exchange experiences and knowledge.

You may successfully chart your trip on the TLC diet and maximize your chances of success by keeping a close eye on your progress, evaluating your food and lifestyle choices, paying attention to your body, and making the required adjustments. It's crucial to be proactive, persistent, and patient in your attempts to improve your cardiovascular health and lower your cholesterol levels because progress may take some time.

Summary

To sum up, the TLC (Therapeutic Lifestyle Changes) diet provides a whole strategy for raising physical activity, changing eating, and modifying lifestyle in order to improve cardiovascular health and lower cholesterol levels. People can improve their general health and lower their risk of heart disease, stroke, and other cardiovascular disorders by adhering to the TLC diet's principles.

We've covered a lot of ground in this article on the TLC diet, including meal plans, physical activity suggestions, nutritional requirements, and social situational awareness techniques. We've also talked about how crucial it is to keep an eye on things, adapt as necessary, and ask for help from medical professionals and encouraging groups.

The TLC diet requires commitment, perseverance, and a readiness to make long-term lifestyle adjustments. Your cholesterol levels, cardiovascular health, and general quality of life can all significantly improve if you adopt heart-healthy practices into your daily routine and remain dedicated to your health objectives.

Recall that incremental improvements eventually yield significant outcomes, and any action you take to prioritize your heart health is a positive step in the right direction. Maintain your motivation, knowledge, and connection to your support system and goals as you proceed on the TLC diet's path to improved health.

THE END

www.ingramcontent.com/pod-product-compliance
Lightning Source LLC
Chambersburg PA
CBHW051917250726
48659CB00002B/706